Gastric Bypass Meal Plans

Eating Well After Weight Loss Surgery

By Michelle Border

Gastric Bypass Meal Plans

Eating Well After Weight Loss Surgery

To my Husband,

Through all the *Tough Times* and *Happy Times*

Table of Contents

Introduction

You have made the decision to take control of your health and to get your weight under control. You know that Gastric Bypass Surgery is not going to be easy. No matter what anyone says, this is not taking the easy way out. So before you take the leap, it's time to educate yourself about what kind of meals you will be preparing for yourself through all stages of your recovery.

You will be meeting with a nutritionist who has been assigned by your doctor. Always take the nutritionist's advice first. Because every body is different, you may be given different diet orders than what is written here. This book is to be used primarily for food and menu ideas to get you through your post-op time, without being bored out of your mind.

The first two stages of the gastric bypass diet are not the most enjoyable, but you can still utilize a few tricks to make your food more fun. Just because you have had gastric bypass surgery does not mean that you will have to endure tasteless, bland food for the rest of your life. There are plenty of ways to eat in a delicious, healthful way, and still lose weight.

The Purpose of the Gastric Bypass Recovery Diet

You will be following the four-staged gastric bypass recovery diet in order to help your body heal properly after your surgery. Major abdominal surgery is no joke, so you will have to give your body extra tender loving care to allow for optimal healing. You will have a staple line in your stomach that will need to heal. Your body will require extra protein to repair the tissue in your stomach.

The liquid and pureed parts of the plan are essential for not irritating the staple line. Think of your staples in terms of a wound on the outside of your body. Let's say that you got stitches on your hand after being cut with a knife. The doctor would tell you to protect the wound site by keeping it covered, not allowing it to get irritated, and to not use the injured hand for physical labor.

The same mindset is required for your stomach. The liquid and pureed foods are much gentler, so the stomach will not be required to work as hard. Pureed foods will not be abrasive like solids foods. So, when you get tired of yet another bland protein drink or mug of broth, just remember, you are allowing your stomach to rest and regenerate.

Another primary reason for the gastric bypass diet is to allow your re-sized stomach to grow accustomed to eating smaller amounts of food at once. The actual surgery will reduce your appetite a great deal in the first days and weeks of the surgery. However, once your body starts healing, your brain may want to go back to eating too much food. This is why it is so important to re-train your brain into eating small meals.

You will begin your weight loss journey with the gastric bypass diet. The high protein, low sugar diet is the perfect ways to jump start your efforts. Obviously, you will not lose all of your excess weight during the four stages gastric bypass recovery diet. In most cases, you will continue to lose weight even after you have transitioned back to a more normal diet. But the gastric bypass diet does an excellent job of laying a solid foundation for nutrition that will both feed the body, and allow it to shed excess weight at the same time.

The final reason why you must stick closely to the gastric bypass recovery diet recommendations is so that you avoid potential surgery complications. Some common complications experienced by wayward dieters are: gas, diarrhoea, constipation, nausea and heartburn. The bypass recovery diet is designed to keep these discomforts to an absolute minimum. So, you will be doing yourself and your digestive tract a huge favor by sticking to it.

Stage One of the Gastric Bypass Post Surgery Diet

Stage one of the diet is clear, sugar-free, fat-free liquids. You will begin drinking as soon after your surgery as you are able. Your choices for this part of your diet are rather limited, however, it will only last three to seven days, depending on your doctor's orders. The good news is that you will drop a lot of weight during these first days.

Your goal will be to drink approximately four ounces of clear liquid every hour for 12-16 hours, or 42 to 70 ounces per day. A lot of patients find it helpful to use a shot glass or medicine cup to measure the liquid and set a timer for every fifteen minutes. Remember to sip your liquid slowly and stop if you start to feel full.

Acceptable liquids for phase one:

-unsweetened clear juices including: light apple, light white grape, light cranberry

-diluted regular juice, 50/50 with water

-sugar free gelatin

-sugar free popsicles (no fruit added)

-fat-free chicken or beef broth

-decaf tea including herbal tea

-non-carbonated 0 calorie flavored drinks (Crystal Light or Fruit 2 O)

MICHELLE BORDER

Stage Two of the Gastric Bypass Post Surgery Diet

Once you have received the all-clear from your doctor, it is time to proceed onto stage two. Stage two is the full liquid part of the diet. You will be adding in milk products (including yogurt!) and protein drinks now. This is where you will begin paying very close attention to your protein intake. You will be aiming for 40-60 grams of protein each day. You will need to continue drinking 42-70 ounces of liquid each day.

You have many protein drink choices, some of the more well-known brands are:

> ➢ Carnation instant breakfast and skim milk

> ➢ Boost

> ➢ Ensure

> ➢ EAS

> ➢ Isomer

> ➢ Spiru-tein

> ➢ Designer Whey

> ➢ Carb Solutions

You may feel free to use another brand of protein drink as long as it does not contain more than 15-20 grams of sugar, and has a minimum of 13 grams of protein per eight ounces.

You will continue to drink small amounts throughout the day, 1-2 ounces every 15 minutes will keep you on track. If you are feeling full, stop. Stage two generally lasts for about three weeks, but you will need to wait for your doctor to give permission to move onto stage three.

Stage Three of the Gastric Bypass Post Surgery Diet

By the time you have reached stage three of the post surgery diet, you should be craving some food with flavor and a bit of texture. You have been drinking everything, and everything you have been drinking has been thin and probably tasted like protein powder. You will not be going hog-wild during this stage, or any stage for that matter, but you can start to experiment with ingredients now.

Stage three is made up of pureed foods and liquids. You still want to have everything made into a smooth texture, but this can easily be accomplished by blending your food in a food processor. Purchasing a few appliances will make your life much easier, so I recommend that you buy at least one of these, but preferably both of them.

The first tool you will need, and also the most versatile is the Cuisinart Mini Prep Food Processor.

You will be able to puree single servings, or a few servings at once using this tool, and it cleans up quickly and easily. You can do foods with a thicker consistency like chicken salad, or thin soups. If you only buy one tool, get this one.

A second tool that I find essential is the Magic Bullet. You will use your magic bullet for smoothies, protein shakes, and for pureeing soups and stews. If you go ahead and invest the money in these tools you will not become frustrated with a lack of choices in Stage 3 later on.

You can take most meals and turn them into a good Stage 3 meal, as long as they are not high in fat and sugar. Remember, you are still dieting in this stage, so you need to be making the best choices.

How Should You Be Eating During Stage Three?

Obviously, all of your foods will be pureed. Why? Well, if you eat food that is in chunks, you could block the exit of your stomach. You can begin eating three meals a day now, as opposed to a bit every hour, but remember, you are still keeping your portions small. You are in the process of re-training your brain to stop eating before you become full. Learning this skill quickly will serve you better for long term weight loss success.

Take your time and eat slowly. Savor each bite of food you put into your mouth and think about what you are eating. Never eat anywhere but the table. Eating while you are distracted may cause you to over-eat.

When you sit down to begin your meal, remember to eat your high protein foods first. You want to make sure to get them in before you start feeling full. Protein first, fruits and vegetables second, carbohydrates last. Protein is the most important because it helps your body continue to heal, and it also helps you to stay satisfied for longer periods of time.

Continue to drink water, at least 42 ounces daily, but remember to drink in small amounts. Do not drink while you are having a meal, this might overfill your stomach. Instead, drink at least 30 minutes prior to eating, and wait around 45 minutes after the meal has finished to resume drinking.

What Foods Can You Enjoy?

As I mentioned earlier, protein is the most essential part of your meal. You will be choosing lean proteins here. Pureed chicken, fish, and turkey are good staples to keep in the house. Just make sure that these are lean cuts and are trimmed of fat and cooked without skin. Cans or pouches of tuna and salmon are great to keep on hand. They are already cooked, so you can just pop the can open, puree it for a few seconds and eat.

Soft scrambled eggs, egg whites or Egg Beaters may all be used, just remember to whiz them through your food processor first. Your food must have a smooth consistency, or you risk it getting stuck. Cook your eggs with a spray of Pam, not butter, and feel free to add some low fat or fat free cheese.

You can also get your much-needed protein from dairy products. Light Ricotta Cheese, and Fat Free Cottage cheese are low in calories and fat, and high in protein. Smooth yogurts, without chunks of fruit are permitted, as well as greek yogurt. Choose greek yogurt as often as possible, it contains about twice as much protein as regular yogurt.

Foods that should be avoided include fatty cuts of meat, canned chicken or fish packed in oil, hotdogs, lunch meats, beef, and fatty cheeses.

Fruits and vegetables should be included in your diet, but pay close attention to which kind you are eating. Always eat your vegetables cooked, they are easier to digest this way. Stay away from the vegetables notorious for causing gas like broccoli, cauliflower, cabbage and onions. Your fruits also need to be cooked. Canned fruit is good because it is already cooked, but it needs to be packed in water, fruit juice, or very light syrup. Drain off the syrup or fruit juice before pureeing.

If you enjoy hot cereals, you can eat Cream of Wheat or unflavored grits. Both may be flavored with some cinnamon and stevia, or an artificial sweetener.

Quantity Counts

Remember, your newly-sized stomach will not be able to hold a lot of food at once. At this point, it will only be able to hold about 3-4 tablespoons at one time. So, when you are planning your meals, you will eat 2 to 3 tablespoons of protein, and half a tablespoon, up to 1 full tablespoon of fruit, veggies or hot cereal. You will be stretching your meal time out over 15-30 minutes. Eat very slowly.

If you are full before you have finished your 3-4 tablespoons, stop! Do not continue eating when you are full. Remember, the goal is to learn to stop **before** you feel full. This is why it is absolutely essential that you eat your protein first.

MICHELLE BORDER

Meal Plans for Stage 3

Monday

Breakfast: Peaches and Cream Protein Shake *(Recipe in next Chapter)*
Cream of Wheat Cereal

Lunch: Chicken Salad *(Recipe in next Chapter)*
Pureed Steamed Carrots

Dinner: Pureed Turkey
Pureed Sweet Potato with Cinnamon and Stevia

Tuesday

Breakfast: Soft Scrambled Egg Beaters
Unsweetened Applesauce

Lunch: Pureed Cottage Cheese w/ Pureed Canned Peaches

Dinner: Salmon Salad *(Recipe in next Chapter)*
Pureed Acorn Squash with Stevia and Cinnamon

Wednesday

Breakfast: Chocolate Ricotta Crème *(Recipe in next Chapter)*
Cream of Wheat

Lunch: Favorite Canned Soup, Pureed

Dinner: Pureed Turkey
Pureed Mashed Potatoes *(Recipe in next Chapter)*

Thursday

Breakfast: Apples and Cinnamon Protein Shake *(Recipe in next Chapter)*

Lunch: Chicken Salad *(Recipe in next Chapter)*
Pureed Steamed Spinach with a Sprinkle of Parmesan Cheese

Dinner: Crab Salad *(Recipe in next Chapter)*
Pureed Tomatoes

Friday

Breakfast: Pureed Cottage Cheese with Pureed Peaches

Lunch: Tuna Salad *(Recipe in next Chapter)*
Steamed Carrots

Dinner: Italian Chicken *(Recipe in next Chapter)*
Pureed Italian Zucchini *(Recipe in next Chapter)*

Saturday

Breakfast: Greek Yogurt Sweetened with Stevia
Unsweetened Applesauce

Lunch: Chocolate Ricotta Crème *(Recipe in next Chapter)*
Pureed Canned Pears

Dinner: Pureed Turkey
Pureed Steamed Sweet Potato with Cinnamon and Stevia

Sunday

Breakfast: Pureed Cottage Cheese with Stage 1 Baby Food Plums

Lunch: Salmon Salad *(Recipe in next Chapter)* Unsweetened Applesauce

Dinner: Pureed Chicken
Pureed Mashed Potatoes *(Recipe in next Chapter)*

Freezer Cooking Frees Up Your Time

Before I give you all of my delicious Stage 3 diet recipes, I want to offer up some advice. The recipes will yield way more than one portion. Remember, each portion will only be 1-3 tablespoons. Instead of just tossing out the leftovers, or instead of eating the same thing for five or six meals in a row, put the leftovers in the freezer instead.

All you will need is a tablespoon measuring spoon and a few ice cube trays. After you have prepared a recipe, measure out what you will be eating for that meal. After you have eaten your meal, measure out the remaining food into the appropriate portion into an ice cube section. For your proteins, you will measure 2-3 tablespoons of your protein foods, and ½ to 1 tablespoon of your fruits, veggies, and Cream of Wheat.

Allow the food to freeze for about 4-5 hours, then you can take the cubes out of the trays and put them into a labeled zip top bag. When you are ready to eat the same meal again, simply thaw out a cube at room temperature, or you could pop it into the microwave for 10-30 seconds, depending on your microwave.

Recipes for Stage 3

Peaches and Cream Protein Shake

1 scoop of vanilla protein powder
½ cup skim milk
2 tablespoons pureed canned peaches
2 ice cubes

In your Magic Bullet, pour in the milk first, then add protein powder, peaches, and ice cubes. Blend until smooth.

This recipe makes more 2-3 servings. A serving is 3-4 tablespoons.

Chicken Salad

One can of chicken breast
1-2 tablespoons of fat free mayo
1/8 teaspoon sea salt
1/8 teaspoon Mrs. Dash

Place all ingredients in your mini food processor, blend until smooth, season to taste. One serving is 2-3 tablespoons.

Salmon Salad

One can of salmon packed in water
1-2 tablespoons of fat free mayo
1/8 teaspoon sea salt
1/8 teaspoon Mrs. Dash

Place all ingredients in your mini food
processor, blend until smooth, season to
taste. One serving is 2-3 tablespoons.

Chocolate Ricotta Crème

½ cup of part skim ricotta
½ teaspoon unsweetened cocoa powder
¼ teaspoon vanilla extract
1 packet of stevia or artificial sweetener

Place all ingredients into your mini food
processor. Blend until well mixed. You can
add more or less stevia according to your
taste preference. One serving is 2-3
tablespoons.

Tuna Salad

One can of tuna packed in water
1-2 tablespoons of fat free mayo
1/8 teaspoon sea salt
1/8 teaspoon Mrs. Dash

Place all ingredients in your mini food processor, blend until smooth, season to taste. One serving is 2-3 tablespoons.

Apples And Cinnamon Protein Shake

1 scoop of vanilla protein powder
½ cup skim milk
2 tablespoons unsweetened applesauce
¼ teaspoon cinnamon
1 packet of stevia
2 ice cubes

In your Magic Bullet, pour in the milk first, then add protein powder, applesauce, cinnamon and stevia, and ice cubes. Blend until smooth. Adjust the seasonings to your taste. You may prefer it without the stevia. A serving is 3-4 tablespoons.

Mashed Potatoes

1 yukon gold potato
¼ cup skim milk
salt
pepper

Peel the potato, cut into 2 inch chunks. Place potato chunk into boiling water and cook 15-20 minutes until they are fork tender. Place cooked potatoes into your mini food processor, add milk, salt and pepper. Blend until smooth. Taste the potatoes and adjust seasonings to your taste.
The serving size is ½ to 1 tablespoon.

Crab Salad

One can of crab packed in water
1-2 tablespoons of fat free mayo
1/8 teaspoon sea salt
½ a packet of stevia

Place all ingredients in your mini food processor, blend until smooth, season to taste. You may want to add more stevia, depending on how sweet you like your crab salad. One serving is 2-3 tablespoons.

Italian Chicken

1 chicken breast
1/8 teaspoon dried oregano
1/8 teaspoon dried basil
1/8 teaspoon garlic
1 teaspoon parmesan cheese
1 tablespoon of water

Place all ingredients into your mini food processor. Blend until smooth. You may need to add more or less water to get a nice, smooth consistency.

The serving size is 2-3 tablespoons.

Italian Zucchini

1 zucchini
1/8 teaspoon basil
1/8 teaspoon oregano
1/8 teaspoon garlic
1 teaspoon parmesan cheese

Place all ingredients into you mini food processor. Blend until smooth.

The serving size is 1 tablespoon.

Now remember, as long as it is okay with your doctor and nutritionist, you can experiment with pureeing other prepared foods, as long as they are low in fat, low in sugar, and do not contain any of the vegetables that are likely to give you gas (broccoli, cauliflower, cabbage, celery, etc.)

MICHELLE BORDER

Stage 4 of the Gastric Bypass Post Surgery Diet

Stage 4 will begin approximately eight weeks after your surgery, but your doctor and nutritionist will have a more firm date for you. This is when you finally get to introduce some foods with some texture. Stage 4 is also known as the soft foods diet. Soft foods are defined as any foods that are very easy to chew. Foods like scrambled eggs, well cooked veggies, lean ground turkey, cooked or canned fruit, a ripe banana, etc. In my opinion, the best part about this stage of the diet was getting to add in I Can't Believe It's Not Butter Spray. I love that stuff!

You finally get to add texture back into your diet, but make sure not to take it overboard. Your food still needs to be very soft and easy to chew. It is also your job to ensure that your food is so well chewed that there are absolutely no lumps or chunks left when you swallow. Did I make that clear enough?

Your primary job is to think about every single bite you take. Chew it at least 20-30 times, and then swallow.

You will continue to only drink water in

between your meals. Take your last drink at least 30 minutes before your meal, and do not resume drinking until 45 minutes have passed after your meal. You should now be aiming to drink between 4 and 8 ounces every hour. Your daily water intake should now be in the 42-60 ounces per day range.

Just because you have added texture back into your diet does not mean that you get to go crazy. You still need to be keeping your diet low fat, low sugar, and most importantly, high in protein. You will always be focusing on protein first when you are eating. Once you have gotten a good serving of protein in, then you can move on to fruits, vegetables, and carbohydrates.

Your stomach has now stretched out some since your surgery so you will be able to eat more at each meal. Most people now have a stomach capacity of about one cup. Remember though, you want to stop eating before you feel full. Chew slowly, and make your meal last between 15 and 30 minutes.

Now is a good time to start implementing

some portion control tricks to make you feel like you are getting more food during your meal times. My favorite meal time mind trick is to eat on a salad plate as opposed to a dinner plate.

The Foods for Stage 4

You will be able to eat all of the foods that were eaten in stage four, only now, you will not have to run them through your food processor. If it is low in fat and low in sugar, and you can cook it into a soft consistency, it's fair game.

Avoid these foods for the next few months until your doctor has given you the green light:

- Nuts and seeds
- Popcorn
- Dried fruits
- Sodas
- High fiber, gassy veggies
- Tough or dry meat
- Bread

Your protein selections should include chicken, turkey, fish (canned and fresh), ricotta and cottage cheese, other low fat cheeses, skim milk, and tofu.

Your vegetable selections are the same as in stage three. You can have any cooked vegetable, except for the vegetables that are likely to cause gas (broccoli, cauliflower, cabbage, onions). You vegetables should be steamed, canned or boiled until they are soft enough to mash with your fork. You may also include potatoes, sweet potatoes and yams.

Fruits are a delicious way to add a bit more flavor to your diet. Stick to cooked or canned fruits. Canned peaches, pears, apples, pineapple, and mandarin oranges are all great choices, just make sure they are packed in juice or water, not syrup. A ripe banana is the only fruit that you may eat raw, but make sure that it is soft enough to mash with a fork.

Your stomach has now stretched out some since your surgery so you will be able to eat more at each meal. Most people now have a stomach capacity of about one cup.

MICHELLE BORDER

Meal Plan for Stage 4

Monday

Breakfast- Pina Colada Protein Shake*(Recipe in next Chapter)*
Lunch- Turkey Chili *(Recipe in next Chapter)*

Dinner- Poached Salmon with Lemon and Dill *(Recipe in next Chapter)*
Peas

Tuesday

Breakfast- Lemon Ricotta Crème *(Recipe in next Chapter)*
Ripe Banana

Lunch- Stage 4 Chicken Salad *(Recipe in next Chapter)*

Dinner- Fiesta Turkey Burger *(Recipe in next Chapter)*
Baked potato (You will not be eating the skin from the potato, just the inside. You may season it with salt and pepper or Mrs. Dash, and also a few sprays of I Can't Believe It's Not Butter Spray. Use a tablespoon of fat free plain yogurt instead of sour cream)

Wednesday

Breakfast- Poached egg
Roasted Asparagus Tips *(Recipe in next Chapter)*

Lunch- Salmon cakes *(Recipe in next Chapter)*
Canned Mandarin Oranges

Dinner- Ground Turkey in Marinara Sauce
with Spaghetti Squash *(Recipe in next Chapter)*

Thursday

Breakfast- Chocolate Mocha Protein Shake
(Recipe in next Chapter)
Lunch- Pina Colada Ricotta Crème *(Recipe in next Chapter)*

Dinner- Stage 4 Italian Chicken *(Recipe in next Chapter)*
Garlic Mashed Potatoes *(Recipe in next Chapter)*

Friday

Breakfast- Scrambled Eggs with Chicken Sausage
Ripe banana

Lunch- Pumpkin Pie Protein Smoothie
(Recipe in next Chapter)

Dinner- Baked Cod with Lemon and Dill
(Recipe in next Chapter)
Steamed Green Beans with Parmesan Cheese

Saturday

Breakfast- Peach Cobbler Protein Smoothie
(Recipe in next Chapter)

Lunch- Canned Chicken Noodle Soup (choose a low sodium soup)

Dinner- Mexican Ground Turkey *(Recipe in next Chapter)*
Roasted Red Peppers *(Recipe in next Chapter)*

Sunday

Breakfast- Cream of Wheat with Canned Peaches

Lunch- Canned Refried Beans and Low-Fat Cheese

Dinner- Poached chicken
Roasted Sweet Potato Fries *(Recipe in next Chapter)*

Recipes for Stage 4

Pina Colada Protein Shake

1 scoop vanilla protein powder
8 oz. Skim milk
½ cup frozen canned pineapple
1 frozen banana
1/8 teaspoon coconut extract

Pour milk into blender first, then add other ingredients, blend until smooth. One serving is 1 cup of the shake.

Turkey Chili

1 can kidney beans, drained
½ pound of cooked ground turkey
1 large can of diced tomatoes
1 large can of tomato sauce
1-3 teaspoons of chili powder
1-3 teaspoons of cumin

Combine all ingredients in a pot and bring to a boil, simmer for 1-3 hours. 1 serving is 1 cup.

Poached Salmon with Lemon and Dill

¼ cup lemon juice
¼ cup water
1 pound salmon fillet, cut into 2 pieces
¾ teaspoon dill
1 clove of garlic, pressed

Combine the lemon juice and water, heat over medium in a non stick pan until simmering. Add the salmon fillets, then sprinkle the dill on top, followed by the garlic. Bring to a low boil and poach over medium until the salmon is firm, which will be about 10 to 15 minutes.
One serving is about 4 oz.

Lemon Ricotta Crème

½ cup of part skim ricotta
½ teaspoon lemon zest
¼ teaspoon lemon extract
1 packet of stevia or artificial sweetener

Place all ingredients into your mini food processor. Blend until well mixed. You can add more or less stevia according to your taste preference. One serving is ½ to 1 cup.

Stage 4 Chicken Salad

1 can chicken breast packed in water, drained
½ cup mandarin oranges, chopped
1-2 tablespoons of fat free mayo
salt and pepper to taste

Combine all ingredients, the serving size is 1 cup.

Fiesta Turkey Burger

1 pound of ground turkey
½ cup salsa made without onions
1-2 teaspoons cumin
1 teaspoon of chili powder
Combine all ingredients with your hands, then shape into four patties. Cook on the grill or in a skillet until the internal temperature is 180 degrees F. One serving is one patty.

Roasted Asparagus Tips

1 bunch of asparagus
Pam cooking spray
salt and pepper

Heat your oven to 400 degrees. Wash and break off asparagus at the halfway point. Place on a cookie sheet and spray with a few sprays of Pam. Sprinkle with salt and pepper. Bake for 15-20 minutes.

Salmon Cakes

15 oz. Canned salmon
1 egg
2 teaspoons dried parsley
1 ½ teaspoons dijon mustard
½ teaspoon black pepper

Mix ingredients with your hands, form into patties. Place patties on a cookie sheet and bake in a 450 degree oven for 25 minutes, until golden brown on top.

Ground Turkey in Marinara Sauce with Spaghetti Squash

1 pound ground turkey
1 can crushed tomatoes
2 teaspoons basil
2 teaspoons oregano
2 teaspoons of stevia
1 spaghetti squash

Brown turkey meat, then add tomatoes, and herbs, simmer over low for 30 minutes.

Cut the spaghetti squash in half and scrape out the seeds with a spoon. Lay the two halves cut side down in a baking dish and bake at 400 degrees for 45-60 minutes.

Remove the squash from the oven and using a fork, scrape out the spaghetti shaped threads. Dish up ½ cup of spaghetti squash and ½ a cup of sauce, you may sprinkle parmesan cheese on top.

Mocha Protein Shake
1 scoop chocolate protein powder
1 T instant decaf coffee
1 cup skim milk
½ cup ice cubes

Pour milk into the blender first, then add other ingredients, blend until smooth. This recipe makes about 1.5 servings.

Pina Colada Ricotta Crème
½ cup of part skim ricotta
½ cup crushed canned pineapple
½ cup banana slices
¼ teaspoon coconut extract
1 packet of stevia or artificial sweetener

Place all ingredients into your mini food processor. Blend until well mixed. You can add more or less stevia according to your taste preference. One serving is ½ to 1 cup.

Stage 4 Italian Chicken
1 can chicken breast
¼ teaspoon basil
¼ teaspoon oregano
1 tablespoon parmesan cheese

Combine all ingredients, eat at room temperature or heated through. Serving size is ½ to ¾ cup.

Garlic Mashed Potatoes
1 yukon gold potato
1 clove crushed garlic
¼ cup milk
1 tablespoon parmesan cheese

Peel potato and cut into 2 inch segments. Boil potato chunks for 15-20 minutes, until fork tender. Mash with a potato masher and then stir in other ingredients. Add salt and pepper to taste. Serving size is ¼ to ½ a cup.

Pumpkin Pie Protein Smoothie

8 oz. Skim milk
1 scoop of vanilla protein powder
1/4 cup canned pumpkin (freeze this in ice cube trays first)
Dash of pumpkin pie spice

Place milk into the blender first, then the rest of the ingredients. Blend until smooth. Serving size is 1 cup.

Baked Cod With Lemon And Dill

1 Cod fillet
2 tablespoons lemon juice
1/8 teaspoon white pepper
1/8 teaspoon dried dill

Mix lemon juice and herbs. Pour over fish. Spray a baking dish with Pam, then place fish in the dish. Bake in a 350 degree oven for 25-30 minutes, or until the fish flakes with a fork.

Peach Cobbler Protein Smoothie

8 oz. Skim milk
1 scoop of vanilla protein powder
1/4 cup frozen sliced peaches
dash of cinnamon
dash of nutmeg
2-3 ice cubes

Place liquid in the blender first then the rest of the ingredients. Blend until smooth, the serving size is 1 cup.

Mexican Ground Turkey

1 pound ground turkey
1 tablespoon chili powder
1 tablespoon cumin
1 teaspoon garlic powder
1 teaspoon onion powder
¼ teaspoon oregano
¼ to ½ teaspoon of cayenne pepper
1 tablespoon corn starch
½ cup water

Brown turkey in a skillet, add seasonings, stir well, then add water. Simmer on low for 5 minutes. Serving size is ½ to ¾ cup.

Roasted Red Peppers
1 red bell pepper
Pam cooking spray
salt and pepper

Clean and seed a red pepper, and then cut into slices or chunks. Place peppers on a cookie sheet and spray with pam, then salt and pepper. Roast at 400 degrees for 20 minutes. Serving size is ¼ to ½ cup.

Roasted Sweet Potato Fries
1 sweet potato
Pam cooking spray
salt and pepper

Peel the sweet potato, then cut into fries. Place fries on cookie sheet then spray with Pam, then sprinkle with salt and pepper. Roast at 400 degrees for 15 minutes, then remove from oven and toss fries with a spatula. Put fries back in to the over for an additional 10-15 minutes until soft and browned. Serving size is ¼ cup.

Phasing Into Normal Eating

Once you have successfully completed stage 4 of the post surgery diet, you will enter into Stage 5, or normal eating. You will need to complete this stage very gradually, with your nutritionist's assistance. During this last stage, you will slowly be adding in lean red meat, bread, pasta, and rice.

Your protein needs will again increase, 70-90 grams will be your daily target. Your daily water intake should be hitting 60 ounces, and the same rules for drinking water are still important. Drink throughout the day, stop drinking 30 minutes before a meal, and resume drinking 45 minutes after a meal.

Continue to be vigilant in keeping your foods low in fat and sugar, and you should be trained by now to stop eating before you feel full. Remember, you do not want to stretch your stomach out.

By this point, you should have lost a significant amount of weight, and as long as you continue in your good habits, you will continue to lose until you arrive at a healthy weight.

Made in the USA
Middletown, DE
13 January 2021